Table of Contents

Pleural effusion, sometimes referred to as "water on the lungs," is the build-up of excess fluid between the layers of the pleura outside the lungs. The pleura are thin membranes that line the lungs and the inside of the chest cavity and act to lubricate and facilitate breathing. Normally, a small amount of fluid is present in the pleura.

The seriousness of the condition depends on the primary cause of pleural effusion, whether breathing is affected, and whether it can be treated effectively. Causes of pleural effusion that can be effectively treated or controlled include an infection due to a virus, pneumonia or heart failure. Two factors that must be considered are treatment for associated mechanical problems as well as treatment of the underlying cause of the pleural effusion.

BREAKFAST

1. Spicy Aloo Tikki

Prep Time: 10 Minutes

Cook Time: 15 Minutes

Servings: 4

Ingredients

- 2 Tbsp oil
- 1 onion, sliced
- 1/2 tsp coriander seeds
- 1/2 tsp cumin seeds
- 1/2 tsp black peppercorn
- 4 potatoes (boiled), mashed
- 1/2 cup peas (boiled), mashed
- 1 cup ginger paste
- 1/2 tsp salt
- 1 tsp red chilli powder
- Ground spice
- 1 Green chilli

- 1/2 cup coriander leaves
- 1/2 tsp maida
- for garnishing curd
- for garnishing mint chutney

Instructions

1. Heat oil in a pan.
2. Add sliced onion to it and fry till golden brown.
3. In another pan, dry roast coriander seeds, cumin seeds and black peppercorn for a while. Grind them together.
4. Take mashed potatoes in a bowl along with mashed peas.
5. Add ginger paste followed by fried onion and mix them thoroughly.
6. Now add salt, red chilli powder, ground spice, green chilli and coriander leaves.
7. Mix these ingredients well to make a sticky mixture.
8. Add maida to the bowl and mix again.
9. Now, make round balls for tikki out of the mixture and refrigerate for 30 minutes.
10. After refrigeration, pan fry the tikkis in some oil till golden brown.

11. Serve hot and crispy Aloo tikki garnished with curd
    and mint chutney.

Prep Time: 10 Minutes

Cook Time: 20 Minutes

Servings: 2

Ingredients

- 2 Tbsp Oil
- 1 tsp Mustard seeds
- 1 tsp Cumin seeds
- 1 tsp Peanuts
- 1/2 tsp Sesame seeds
- 1 tsp Urad dal
- 7-8 Nos Curry leaves
- 11-12 Nos Cashewnuts
- 1 Nos Onion, chopped
- 1/4 Cup Carrot, chopped
- 1/4 Cup Beans, chopped
- 1/4 Cup Peas
- 1 tsp Ginger
- 1 Nos Green chilli
- 1 tsp Salt
- 1/2 tsp Turmeric powder

- 1 Cup Vermicelli
- 1 Cup Water

Instructions

1. Heat oil in a pan.
2. Add mustard seeds, cumin seeds, peanuts, sesame seeds, urad dal, curry leaves and cashew nuts.
3. Saute them for a while and add onion. Mix thoroughly.
4. Add chopped carrot and beans along with peas, ginger and green chilli. Mix well.
5. Add salt and turmeric powder and mix until yellowish in colour.
6. Slowly pour vermicelli in the pan.
7. Stir slowly, adding water as required.
8. Cover the pan for a while to let it cook on a medium flame.
9. Remove the lid and check if the water has evaporated.
10. Semiya Upma is ready to serve hot.

Prep Time: 10 Minutes

Cook Time: 20 Minutes

Servings: 2

Ingredients

- 1 Cup Besan
- 1/2 tsp Salt
- 1 tsp Black Pepper
- 1 Onion, chopped
- 1/2 Cup Paneer, grated
- 1 Tomato
- 2 Green Chillies
- 1/2 tsp Ajwain
- 1/2 Cup Coriander Leaves
- 1 Cup Water

Instructions

1. Take besan in a bowl, add salt, black pepper, onion, grated paneer, tomato, green chillies, ajwain and coriander leaves.

2. Whisk all the ingredients together in the bowl along with water to make a mixture.

3. Add more water to make its consistency light.

4. Now take a pan and put some amount of the besan mixture to pan fry it.

5. Fry till it turns solid, crispy and golden brown.

6. Put some grated paneer, onion, black pepper and coriander leaves over.

7. Fold it and serve hot with red chilli chutney.

Prep Time: 10 Minutes

Cook Time: 15 Minutes

Servings: 2

Ingredients

For salad:

- 1 cup Rocket leaves
- 1/3 cup Lollo rosso leaves
- 1 cup Corn kernels
- 1 cup Lettuce leaves
- 1/3 cup Spring onions
- 1/2 cup Sprouted chickpeas
- 1/2 cup Cranberries
- 1 medium Sweet potatoes (cooked)
- 1 cup Carrots, grated
- 1/3 cup Feta cheese
- to taste Salt
- A pinch of Cumin-fennel powder (optional), roasted

For dressing:

- 1/2 cup Cranberries

- 2 tbsp Olive oil
- to taste Salt and Pepper
- 1/3 cup Spring onion, sliced
- 2 tbsp Balsamic vinegar
- 1 tbsp Maple syrup

For garnishing:

- to taste Pepper
- Few Cranberries

Instructions

1. Toss all the ingredients for the salad in a bowl.
2. Take all the ingredients of the dressing and blend.
3. Toss the salad with the dressing.
4. Serve garnished with black pepper and dried cranberries.

Prep Time: 10 Minutes

Cook Time: 15 Minutes

Servings: 2

Ingredients

- 2 tsp oil
- 3 tsp butter
- 1 tsp garlic
- 2 tsp green Chillies
- 2 tsp ginger
- 6-7 Curry Leaves
- 1/2 cup onion, chopped
- 3 tsp salt
- 2 tsp turmeric powder
- 2 tsp chilli powder
- 1 1/2 tsp pav bhaji masala
- 1 tsp coriander stems
- 1/2 cup tomatoes, chopped
- 4 Eggs
- Coriander leaves

Instructions

1. Take a pan and pour oil in it.

2. Add butter, garlic, green chillies and ginger to the pan.

3. Stir them well until golden brown.

4. Now mix curry leaves and chopped onions to the pan and saute together.

5. Add salt, turmeric powder, chilli powder, Pav bhaji masala and mix them well.

6. Top it with Coriander stems and chopped tomatoes and mix it in the pan along with other ingredients.

7. Now add the eggs to the pan and whisk them thoroughly until cooked.

8. Pour some butter over and garnish it with coriander leaves.

9. Serve hot with buttered bread.

Prep Time: 10 Minutes

Cook Time: 25 Minutes

Servings: 2

Ingredients

- 6-8 eggs
- 5-6 sausages
- 1 chicken ham
- 1-2 onions
- 1/4th red bell pepper
- Olive oil
- 3-4 Tbsp butter
- 1 potato
- 2 green chillies
- 1 cup mushrooms

Instructions

1. Slice up sausages, ham, red bell pepper and chillis.
2. Heat olive oil and butter. Add onions and saute them. Then add small chopped peices of potatoes.

3. Add the sausages, ham, chillies, bell peppers and diced mushrooms. Cook for few minutes.

4. Add salt and pepper and keep them aside.

5. In a seperate bowl, whisk the eggs with some salt and pepper. Make the batter fluffy/frothy.

6. In another bowl, add butter and put the sausage mixture in it.

7. Add the eggs and put them in the oven for 5-7 minutes at 170-180 degree.

8. Serve the frittata in a plate. Garnish with coriander and sprouts and serve.

Prep Time: 05 Minutes

Cook Time: 30 Minutes

Servings: 2

Ingredients

- 1 bowl leftover pasta
- 1 red pepper
- 2-3 mushrooms
- 1 multigrain bread loaf
- 50 gram mozzarella cheese
- 10-12 olives
- to taste butter
- to taste salt & pepper
- 3 tsp extra virgin olive oil

Instructions

1. Slice the red pepper in half, deseed and julienne.
2. Julienne the mushrooms.
3. Slice the bread loaf in 2 thick slices.
4. In a hot pan add 2-3 tsp olive oil.

5. Add red pepper, mushrooms and salt to taste.

6. Add 4-5 olives halved.

7. Now gently saute the vegetables.

8. Add the leftover pasta, cook for some time, till the pasta is heated.

9. Transfer the pasta mixture to a bowl.

10. Butter the bread slices generously.

11. Slice mozzarella cheese and put it on one of the bread slices.

12. Scoop the pasta onto the bread slice.

13. Add one more mozzarella slice on top and cover with the other slice of bread.

14. Heat the pan and add few drops of olive oil.

15. Toast the bread till both sides turns golden brown.

16. Serve it hot.

Prep Time: 05 Minutes

Cook Time: 30 Minutes

Servings: 2

Ingredients

For french toast:

- 2 eggs
- 2 tsp sugar
- Vanilla essence (to flavour)
- 1 cup milk
- 4 pcs bread
- 50 gms butter
- for garnishing honey
- to taste frozen blue berries

For musk melon salad:

- 1 musk melon
- 250 gms red and green grapes
- to taste frozen strawberries
- to taste mint leaves
- 50 gms walnuts

- 1 tsp pumpkin seeds

- Honey (to drizzle)

- 1 tsp olive oil

Instructions

1. Prepare the French toast:

2. Break the eggs into bowl and whisk a little.

3. Add 2 tsp of sugar, some vanilla essence and 1 small cup of milk. Whisk to make the egg wash.

4. In a hot pan add some butter. Dip the pieces of bread in the egg wash and put them in the pan. Add some egg wash on top.

5. Fry till the pieces of bread are golden brown.

6. For the final plating put some berries and drizzle honey to garnish.

7. Prepare the musk melon salad:

8. Take a musk melon, cut in half.

9. Scoop the musk melon from the middle, after discarding the seeds put the pulp in a bowl.

10. Half the red and green grapes and put them in a bowl. Put some frozen strawberries

11. Add some mint leaves. Add chopped walnuts, pumpkin seeds. Drizzle some honey.

12. Add a teaspoon of olive oil and mix.

13. Serve in the musk melon shell.

Prep Time: 10 Minutes

Cook Time: 30 Minutes

Servings: 2

Ingredients

- 4-6 Tbsp oil
- 1/2 tsp skinned urad dal
- 1/4 tsp mustard seeds
- 1/4 tsp cumin seeds
- 2 sliced onions
- 4-5 curry leaves
- 3-4 chopped green chillies
- 2 tsp garlic paste
- 1 tsp ginger paste
- 2 tsp ground coconut
- Turmeric powder, a pinch
- Salt
- 250 gm of diced vegetables
- 1 chopped tomato
- 150 gm semolina
- 250 ml hot water

- 100 ml curd
- 2 Tbsp chopped coriander
- Juice 1 lime

Instructions

1. Heat oil, fry dal, mustard and cumin seeds for 15 seconds.
2. Add onions, curry leaves, chopped chillies, ginger, garlic, turmeric, and salt and coconut paste. Stir and fry for 5 minutes.
3. Add vegetables and tomato. Fry for 3-4 minutes.
4. Add semolina. After 2-3 minute, pour in water and curd. Cook for 5 minutes until dry.
5. Garnish with coriander and sharpen with lemon juice.
6. Serve hot with rasam.

Prep Time: 10 Minutes

Cook Time: 30 Minutes

Servings: 2

Ingredients

For chicken stuffing:

- 2 tsp olive oil
- 1/2 tsp garlic
- 1 tsp chopped onion
- 3/4 tsp chopped celery
- 80 gm chopped chicken
- 3/4 tsp green chilly
- 3/4 vegetable stock
- 2 tsp soya sauce

For sauteed mushrooms:

- 1 tsp butter
- 1 tsp garlic
- 1/2 cup mushroom
- 3/4 glass vegetable stock
- 1 tsp basil

- Pinch of salt

- Pepper powder

For egg white omelette:

- 1 tsp oil

- 3 egg whites

Instructions

For the chicken filling:

1. Saute garlic, onion and celery in olive oil.

2. Add small pieces of chicken, green chilly and pour vegetable stock for flavor and saute them all together for 10 minutes.

3. Add soya sauce and avoid using salt. Saute them all together till it gets dry.

4. For sauteed mushrooms:

5. Saute butter and garlic in the pan.

6. Add mushroom and vegetable stock for flavor. Saute them all together.

7. Add basil and pinch of salt for taste.

8. Add little pepper for punch and saute them all together till it gets ready to eat.

9. Presentation:

10. Pour olive oil in the pan and put the egg white in it.

11. Let it cook for sometime and then put the chicken filling on top of it and roll it from both the side.

Prep Time: 10 Minutes

Cook Time: 45 Minutes

Servings: 4

Ingredients

- 750 gm chicken
- One pod of garlic
- 1/2 tsp coriander seeds
- 1/2 tsp ginger-finely chopped
- 2 Tbsp garlic paste
- 7 small onions-finely chopped
- 6 whole red chillies
- 5 cloves
- 1/2 tsp aniseed
- 2 sticks of cinnamon
- 100 gm khoya
- 250 gm yogurt
- 2 cooking spoons of clarified butter
- Salt according to taste

Instructions

1. Mix all the ingredients except for the chicken, cloves, cardamom and the cinnamon with the yogurt and keep ready.
2. Heat the clarified butter and add the cloves, cardamom and cinnamon.
3. Add all the ingredients except for the chicken and stir till the masalas is done.
4. Add the chicken and cook till its done.
5. Do not add any water.

11. Roasted Chicken with Mushroom and Wine Sauce

Prep Time: 10 Minutes

Cook Time: 45 Minutes

Servings: 4

Ingredients

- 1 chicken- whole, with skin
- 2 tsp butter
- 1 glass white wine
- 150 ml chicken stock
- 1 tbsp oil
- 1 tbsp spring onion paste
- 1 tsp garlic paste
- 1/2 tsp basil
- 200 gms mushrooms, sliced
- Salt and pepper
- 1 tbsp tomato puree
- 3 tbsp lemon juice
- 2 tbsp herbs, chopped
- 1 tbsp cream

- Garnish: Roasted walnuts, chopped

Instructions

1. Place chicken in a roasting tin.
2. Cover chicken breast with butter.
3. Pour over the wine and stock. Roast at 220 degree C for 1 hour or until the chicken is tender and colored. Cool.
4. Heat oil. Saute spring onions, garlic and basil for 1 minute.
5. Stir in the mushrooms, wine, seasoning and tomato puree.
6. Reduce over a high flame until the wine evaporates. Cool.
7. Stir in lemon juice, herbs and cream.
8. Whisk in the juices without any fat from the roasting tin. Carve the chicken.
9. Spoon over dressing and garnish with an extra helping of herbs and chopped walnuts.

Prep Time: 10 Minutes

Cook Time: 45 Minutes

Servings: 4

Ingredients

For paste of gravy/sauce:

- 2 tbsp oil
- 1 tsp ginger paste
- 1 tsp garlic paste
- 1 cup onion, chopped
- 1 cup tomato, chopped
- 3/4 cup coconut, grated

To make gravy/sauce (Kat in Marathi):

- 3 tbsp oil
- spice paste (as above)
- to taste salt
- 1 tsp red chilli paste
- 1 tsp garam masala
- 1/2 tsp turmeric powder
- 1 tsp cumin-coriander powder

- 1/2 tsp cinnamon & clove powder
- 3 cups water (or as required to adjust the consistency)

To make usal:

- 3 tbsp oil
- 1 tsp garlic paste
- 1 tsp ginger paste
- 1/2 tsp hing (asafoetida)
- 1 1/2 cups steamed matki (moth) (soaked overnight)
- 1 cup potato (cut into square pieces), boiled
- 1/2 tsp turmeric powder
- 1 tsp garam masala
- 1/2 tsp cinnamon-clove powder
- 1 lime juice
- 3 cups water (or as required)
- to taste salt

For garnishing:

- onion, chopped
- Mix dry farsan
- coriander, chopped

To serve with:

- Paav, slice of lemon

Instructions

Prepare paste:

1. Heat oil in a pan. Add ginger paste, garlic paste and chopped onion.
2. Saute till the onion is transculent.
3. Now add chopped tomatoes and grated coconut. Mix well and saute it for few minutes.
4. Allow the mixture to cool then grind it into a smooth paste.
5. Prepare gravy/sauce
6. Heat oil in a pan. Add the ready paste into oil and saute it for about 2 minutes.
7. Now add salt, red chilly powder, garam masala, turmeric powder, cumin-coriander powder, clove-cinnamon powder and mix it.
8. Add water and cook till the mixture starts leaving oil.
9. Transfer it in a bowl and keep it aside.

Prepare Usal:

1. Heat oil in a pan. Add ginger paste, garlic paste and asafoetida.
2. Saute it for a minute and add soaked & boiled sprouts along with potatoes. Mix it well.

3. Now add salt, turmeric powder, garam masala, clove-cinnamon powder and lime juice.

4. Add water to it and cook it for about 8-10 minutes.

5. Transfer it in a separate bowl.

Prepare Misal:

1. Take a serving bowl. First pour ready usal in the bowl and then pour the red gravy over it.

2. Thereafter, add finely chopped onion and farsan to the mixture.

3. Garnish it with chopped coriander. Serve it with pav and a slice of lemon

Prep Time: 10 Minutes

Cook Time: 40 Minutes

Servings: 2

Ingredients

- 3 strips of bread - sliced horizontally from a loaf

For the Mint Filling:

- 1 Tbsp blanched spinach paste
- 2 Tbsp mint chutney
- Grated rind 1 lemon
- 100 gm hung curd
- Salt

For the Curry Filling:

- 100 gm hung curd
- 1 tsp prepared mustard
- 1 Tbsp tomato ketchup
- 1 tsp curry powder
- 1 tsp garlic paste
- 1 Tbsp mango chutney

- 1 Tbsp cheese spread
- Salt and pepper

To Finish:

- 100 gm seasoned hung curd
- 2 Tbsp mayonnaise
- 2 tsp butter fresh herbs

Instructions

1. Butter the bread.
2. Combine filling ingredients for mint filling and curry filling.
3. Layer the sandwich with the two fillings.
4. Top with finishing ingredients and serve chilled.

Prep Time: 15 Minutes

Cook Time: 40 Minutes

Servings: 2

Ingredients

- 1 cup brown rice
- 1 green capsicum, large
- 1 onion, medium
- 1 tsp ginger garlic paste
- 30ml curd
- 2 Tbsp coriander mint and green chilli paste
- 1 tsp garam masala
- 1/2 tsp cumin seeds
- 2 bay leaves
- 1/2 tsp coriander powder
- 1 tsp olive oil
- Salt to taste

Instructions

1. In a non-stick vessel, heat oil and add cumin seeds.

2. Once the seeds crackle, add the bay leaves, stir gently and add chopped onions. Cook the onions till they turn brown.

3. Now add ginger garlic paste, coriander mint paste and curd to the vessel and cook well. Once the masala is cooked well, you will start getting a lovely aroma and this is the correct time to stir in the dry masalas.

4. Cook for 5-6 minutes, time to add the crunchy capsicum. Once done, add the rice and 1 1/2 cups of water.

5. Cover the vessel with a lid and let it cook for 15 minutes or till the rice is done.

6. Garnish with some coriander and serve fresh.

Prep Time: 20 Minutes

Cook Time: 1hrs 5 Minutes

Servings: 4

Ingredients

- 1300 Gram zucchini
- 220 grams (Wash few times and soak for 45 minutes) basmati rice
- 15 gram fenugreek (methi)
- 15 gram clarified butter (desi ghee)
- 120 gram clarified butter (desi ghee)
- 4 gram cumin seeds (jeera)
- 1 gram asafoetida (heeng)
- medium green chilles, chopped
- 2 pieces ginger, julienne
- to taste salt

Instructions

1. Wash the Zucchini, Peel and Halve lengthwise. Cut in thin slices.

2. Keep aside.Chop the fresh fenugreek, sprinkle with salt and rub the salt on the leaves with your hands in a bowl.

3. Keep for 5 minutes and wash in running water until all traces of salt have been removed. (This is done to reduce the bitterness of the fenugreek). Shake dry and keep aside.

4. Add clarified butter in a pot. Add cumin seeds, followed by the asafoetida (dissolved in a little water). Then add the fenugreek and increase to medium heat, continue to stir and roast (approx 4-5 minutes) until you can see oil on the sides.

5. Add the Zucchini and stir for a minute, then add green chillies and ginger, stir again. Drain the rice, add to the pot then add salt stirring gently.

6. Cover the pot and leave on slow heat, stirring gently and occasionally for 10-12 minutes or until the rice is fully cooked and moisture is absorbed.Transfer to a bowl and serve.

Prep Time: 20 Minutes

Cook Time: 30 Minutes

Servings: 4

Ingredients

- 1/2 kg mixed vegetables-chopped
- 2 Tbsp yogurt (mix with ginger-garlic paste & leave for 3-4 hours)
- 1 tsp ginger-garlic paste
- 2 tsp lemon juice
- 1 1/2 tsp salt
- 2 Tbsp oil
- 1/2 cup onion-grated

Dry roast separately and grind:

- 1/4 cinnamon
- 1/2 tsp cloves
- 1/4 tsp peppercorns and black cumin
- 1/4 tsp broken up mace
- 1/4 dry grated coconut
- 1 Tbsp coriander seeds

- 1 tsp dagar phool (if easily available)
- 2 Kashmiri mirchi

Instructions

1. Mix the vegetables, yogurt, ginger-garlic paste, lemon juice, salt and grated onions. Keep aside.
2. Heat oil and add the onions and stir-fry till light brown.
3. Add the ground masala, saute till well, mixed and add the vegetable mixture.
4. Bring to a boil, lower the heat, simmer for 3-4 minutes and serve.

Prep Time: 20 Minutes

Cook Time: 30 Minutes

Servings: 4

Ingredients

- 1/2 Kg rajma, boiled
- 2 tbsp olive oil
- 1/2 tsp cumin powder
- 1/2 tsp coriander powder
- 1/2 tsp chili powder
- 1 tsp tabasco
- 2 Lemons
- 1/2 Onion
- Lettuce, chopped
- Processed mozzarella cheese

For salsa sauce:

- 2 Tomatoes
- 1 Onion
- 2 Jalapeno
- 1 Lime

- Handful of coriander leaves
- 1 tsp cumin
- Handful of chives of spring onion
- 4 Corn tortillas
- to taste Salt and pepper

Instructions

Prepare the salsa sauce:

1. Chop tomatoes, onions and jalapenos.
2. In a bowl, add tomatoes, onion, chives of spring onions, jalapenos chopped, and squeeze in 1 lime.
3. Add coriander leaves for the freshness and season it with cumin seeds, salt & pepper and olive oil. Mix them well.
4. Prepare the Burritos:
5. In a pan add olive oil and then heat the pan for a while.
6. Add kidney beans and slightly mash them.
7. Season it with salt and pepper.
8. Add cumin powder, coriander powder, chili powder and let the beans cook for some time.
9. Then add tabasco sauce and squeeze in half a lime to lift the flavors of kidney beans.

10. Chop some onions and add it to kidney beans.

11. In a plate take corn tortilla and add kidney beans mixture, salsa sauce and coriander leaves.

12. Season it with salt.

13. Now fold the tortilla and put it into a baking dish pre sprayed with olive oil.

14. Add a layer of mozzarella cheese and put the baking dish into the oven for 8-10 minutes at 180 degree. Finish with coriander leaves.

Prep Time: 20 Minutes

Cook Time: 45 Minutes

Servings: 2

Ingredients

- 4 medium potatoes - cooked, peeled, and chilled
- 6 Tbsp butter
- 1 large onion - thinly sliced
- Salt - to taste
- Pepper - to taste

Instructions

1. Grate the potatoes thickly. In a pan, melt the butter over medium heat.
2. Add onion and cook until transparent, about five minutes.
3. Add potatoes and stir to blend; press down firmly.
4. Cook over low heat for 25 to 30 minutes, until potatoes are crisp and brown on the bottom.

5. Cut through potatoes from the edge of the pan to center.

6. Carefully run a spatula under cut sections, flipping over one section at a time.

7. Cook until browned.

8. Run spatula under potatoes, loosening them from the skillet.

9. Transfer on to a serving dish, sprinkle with salt and pepper and serve.

Prep Time: 15 Minutes

Cook Time: 20 Minutes

Servings: 2

Ingredients

- 500 Ml Water
- 500 gram Basmati rice
- 100 gram Ghee
- 50 gram Paneer (cooked), chopped
- 100 gram Carrot
- 100 gram Beans
- 100 gram Peas
- 2 small Elaichi
- 2 Cardamoms
- 1 Cinnamon
- 3 Bay leaves
- 2 tbsp Cumin seeds
- 1/2 tbsp Chilli powder
- 1/4 tbsp Turmeric
- to taste Salt
- Coriander leaves

Instructions

1. Heat the ghee and lightly saute all vegetables
2. Add paneer and saute.
3. In a separate pan, saute all spices.
4. Add drained rice and fry for 3 minutes.
5. Add sauteed vegetables and water.
6. Cover and cook until done.
7. Garnish with coriander leaves.

Prep Time: 15 Minutes

Cook Time: 1hrs 20 Minutes

Servings: 6

Ingredients

- 2 potatoes, grated
- A pinch of salt
- Oil, to deep fry

For The Rice:

- 2 cups rice (washed and pre-soaked)
- For the Palak/ Spinach Layer:
- 200 gms spinach (pureed), boiled
- 1 tbsp kasoori methi (pureed with the spinach), boiled
- 2 tbsp ghee
- 3-4 black elaichi daana
- 1/2 stick cinnamon
- 1 tsp jeera
- 1/2 tbsp ginger-garlic paste
- 2 tbsp onion paste
- 1 cup tomato puree

- A pinch of salt

- A pinch of garam masala

For Tomato Paneer Layer:

- 1 tbsp ghee

- 1 tsp jeera

- 1/2 tbsp ginger-garlic paste

- 1 1/2 cups tomato puree

- 1 cup paneer (cubed)

- A pinch of salt

- 1 tsp sugar

- 1/2 tsp garam masala

- 1/4 cup milk

Instructions

For the Aloo Lachchas:

1. Grate the potatoes and soak them in salty water.
2. Drain excess water and deep fry them till golden brown.
3. Drain on an absorbent paper.

For The Rice:

1. Boil the rice with a little salt. Drain water.

2. For the Palak/ Spinach Layer:

3. In a pan add ghee, elaichi dana, cinnamon, jeera and ginger-garlic paste. Saute.

4. Add onion paste. Saute it till golden brown.

5. Add tomato puree. Add garam masala and salt. Cook till it leaves oil on the sides.

6. Add the boiled and pureed spinach-kasoori methi.

7. Cook for 15-20 minutes on medium flame.

For The Tomato Paneer:

1. In a pan add ghee, jeera, ginger-garlic paste.

2. Add tomato puree. Add salt and sugar. Cook till it leaves oil on the sides.

3. Add milk and paneer cubes. Let it cook for 2 minutes on low flame.

4. Plating up:

5. In a baking dish layer the boiled rice.

6. Layer the cooked spinach. Then the rice again.

7. Layer the tomato paneer.

8. Keep layering in this order till the baking dish is full.

9. Add the aloo lachchas and bake for 7-8 minutes at 150 degree C.

10. Serve with a bowl of curd.

21. Amritsari Paneer

Prep Time: 05 Minutes

Cook Time: 20 Minutes

Servings: 6

Ingredients

- 1 Tbsp Refined oil
- 1 tbsp Butter
- 1/2 tbsp Cumin seeds
- 1 piece Casia
- 1 Onion, chopped
- A bit of Ginger, chopped
- 1/2 tbsp Turmeric powder
- 1/2 tbsp Cumin powder
- 1 tsp Coriander powder
- 1 tsp Red chilli powder
- to taste Salt
- 1 Tomato, chopped
- Little bit Sugar
- 2 Green chilies, chopped

- 1/2 tbsp Dry ginger powder
- 200 gram Paneer
- Fresh coriander leaves
- 1/2 Lime

Instructions

1. In a pan, saute refined oil, butter, cumin seeds and casia.
2. Add chopped onion, ginger, turmeric powder, cumin powder, coriander powder, red chili powder and salt to taste. Saute them well together.
3. Add little more water and mix them well
4. Add in chopped tomato, green chilies, dry ginger powder and sugar. Mix them well together.
5. Crumble the paneer over the mixture. Combine them well together.
6. Add butter, fresh coriander leaves and lime.
7. Serve hot .

Prep Time: 15 Minutes

Cook Time: 1hrs 20 Minutes

Servings: 6

Ingredients

- 1 Kg chicken (cut into 10 pieces)

For the powder:

- 1 tbsp black peppercorns
- 1 tbsp fennel (Saunf)
- 1 Cinnamon stick

For the marinade:

- 2 tsp oil
- 2 tbsp spice paste
- 2 tsp red chilli powder
- 2 tsp coriander powder
- to taste salt
- 2 tsp turmeric powder
- 2 tsp pepper-fennel powder
- 3 1/2 tbsp tamarind extract

- 1/2 Lemon (juiced)
- 1 tsp jaggery

For the spice paste:

- 1 tsp red chilli powder
- 1 tsp turmeric powder
- to taste salt
- 1 tsp coriander powder
- 1 tsp cumin powder
- 1 tsp ginger-garlic paste

For the stir fry:

- 1 tsp oil
- 1 onion (diced)
- 1/2 red bell pepper(diced)
- 1 green chilli

Others:

- 2 tsp oil (to sear the chicken)
- for garnishing spring onions with greens
- to garnish for garnishing ginger, julienne
- for garnishing lemon juice

Instructions

Prepare the powder:

- Dry roast black peppercorns, fennel and cinnamon. Grind it in a mortar and pestle.

Prepare the spice paste:

1. Mix all the ingredients together.
2. Prepare the marinade:
3. In a pan add 2 tsp oil and 2 Tbsp spice paste. Saute. Turn off the heat.
4. Add red chilli powder, coriander powder, salt, turmeric powder, pepper-fennel powder, tamarind extract, juice of 1/2 lemon and jaggery.
5. Marinate the chicken with this marinade for 30 minutes.
6. Prepare the stir fry:
7. In a pan add oil.
8. Add onions, bell peppers and green chilli. Saute for 2 minutes. Keep aside.
9. Main preparation:
10. In a pan add oil and sear the chicken from both sides.
11. Add 1-1 1/2 cup water. Cover the pan and cook the chicken for 25-30 minutes.
12. Add the stir fried vegetables. Stir well.

13. Garnish with spring onions, julienne ginger and lemon juice.

14. Serve with steamed rice or paranthas.

Prep Time: 15 Minutes

Cook Time: 20 Minutes

Servings: 4

Ingredients

- 100 gms soya nuggets (soaked in water for 1/2 an hour and drained
- 2 tbsp salt
- 1/2 tbsp garlic paste
- 2 tbsp oil
- 1 cup spring onions, finely chopped
- 2 tbsp green chillies, sliced
- 2 tbsp soya sauce
- 2 tbsp vinegar
- for garnishing Some greens

Instructions

1. Mix together the nuggets, 1 teaspoon salt and garlic paste.

2. Heat the oil, add the onions and stir-fry over high heat till a little brown at the edges.

3. Add the green chillies and stir a few times, add the remaindered salt, soya sauce, vinegar and the nuggets.

4. Stir-fry over high heat for a minute or so and serve garnished with some greens.

Prep Time: 15 Minutes

Cook Time: 1hrs 20 Minutes

Servings: 4

Ingredients

For the Marinade:

- 1/2 kg Chicken
- 1/2 cup Yoghurt
- 25 gram Coriander leaves
- 25 gram Mint leaves
- 10 gram Curry leaves
- 1/2 tsp Cumin seeds
- 1 tsp Coriander seeds
- 1/2 tsp Aniseed powder
- 25 gram Green chillies, chopped
- 20 gram Garlic
- 2 tsp Ginger, chopped
- 1/2 tsp Turmeric powder
- 1 tsp Lime juice
- 1 tsp Poppy seed paste

For main preparation:

- 1 tbsp Clarified butter
- 5-6 Cinnamon pieces
- 1 Bay leaf
- 4-5 Cardamom seeds
- 4-5 Curry leaves
- 4-5 Cloves
- 1 Onion, chopped
- 250 gram Rice (broken)
- 1/2 litre Water

For the masala:

- 2 tbsp Clarified butter
- 5-6 Cinnamon pieces
- 1 Bay leaf
- 4-5 Cloves
- 4-5 Cardamom seeds
- 1 Nutmeg
- 100 gram Onions
- 1 medium Tomato (cut in 4)

Instructions

Prepare the Marinade:

1. Mix yoghurt, coriander leaves, mint leaves, curry leaves, cumin seeds, coriander seeds, aniseed powder, green chillies, garlic, ginger, turmeric powder, lime juice and poppy seed paste and marinate the chicken in it.
2. Keep aside for 1/2 an hour.
3. Prepare the Rice:
4. Heat clarified butter in pan. Add cinnamon, 1 bay leaf, cardamom seeds, curry leaves and cloves. Add onions and saute till they turn translucent and caramelized.
5. Add washed and cleaned rice. Cook till rice turns translucent.
6. Add water. When water comes to a boil, turn flame to low and cover pan.
7. Cook on low flame for at least 15 minutes. The rice is done.

Prepare the Masala:

1. Heat clarified butter in pan and add cinnamon, 1 bay leaf, cardamom seeds, nutmeg and cloves.
2. Add onions and saute till brown. Add tomatoes. Add marinated chicken.

3. Cover pan and cook for at least 5 minutes on a medium flame. Remove cover and cook on low flame for another 10 minutes to allow gravy to thicken.

4. Layer the serving bowl with alternating layers of rice and the chicken masala.

5. Garnish the top with a boiled egg cut in four pieces, roasted cashews and raisins.

Prep Time: 10 Minutes

Cook Time: 30 Minutes

Servings: 1

Ingredients

- 1 cup refined oil
- 1 egg
- 2 tbsp vinegar
- 1/2 tsp sugar
- Salt - to taste
- 1/4 tsp black pepper powder
- 1/4 tsp mustard powder or mustard oil

For Submarine Sandwich:

- 1 French loaf (12 inches)
- 3-4 tbsp mayonnaise or olive oil
- 4 salami slices
- 4 ham slices
- 2 cheese slices
- 4 thinly sliced onions
- Dried oregano - to taste

- Mustard sauce - to taste
- Lettuce leaves (optional)

Instructions

1. Break the egg and put it in the blender.
2. Add the vinegar, salt, pepper, mustard and sugar.
3. Switch on the blender at full speed and simultaneously start pouring the oil in a thin stream through the small opening on top of the blender till it thickens to the required consistency.
4. For Subamarine Sandwiches:
5. Slit the bread horizontally leaving it joined on one side.
6. Spread the mayonnaise on the side or you could drizzle generous amounts of olive oil instead of mayonnaise.
7. Arrange the ham, salami and cheese slices over this.
8. Put the onions on top of this, spread a bit of mustard sauce and sprinkle the oregano.
9. Fold the other half of the bread over and serve.

26. Chicken Fried Rice

Prep Time: 10 Minutes

Cook Time: 30 Minutes

Servings: 2

Ingredients

- 1 Cup rice
- 1 tbsp salt
- oil
- 2 tsp garlic paste
- 1 cup spring onions, finely chopped
- 3/4 cup chicken (cooked), finely chopped
- 2 tbsp celery , finely chopped
- 2 tsp soya sauce
- 1 tbsp vinegar
- 1 tsp chilli sauce

Instructions

1. Boil the rice with 1 tsp salt and 1 Tbsp oil, till 'bite-like'.
2. Drain and rinse under cold water.

3. Leave in the colander and work 1 Tbsp oil into it.

4. Heat the rest of the oil and saute the garlic and onions, till onions are a light brown.

5. Add the chicken and stir-fry till well mixed.

6. Add the soya sauce, vinegar and chilli sauce, mix well and add the rice.

7. Stir till rice and chicken are well mixed and serve.

27. Vegetable Fried Rice

Prep Time: 10 Minutes

Cook Time: 20 Minutes

Servings: 4

Ingredients

- 1 bowl rice (A day old rice make the best fried rice), boiled
- 1 tbsp oil
- 2-3 garlic cloves, chopped
- 1 red chilli, chopped
- 1 tbsp carrots, chopped
- 3-4 baby corn, chopped
- 4-5 tbsp cabbage (diced)
- 1/2 tbsp sesame oil
- 4-5 green beans, chopped
- to taste salt
- Pepper
- 1 tsp soy sauce
- 2-3 tbsp wine (optional)
- for garnishing spring onion greens

Instructions

1. In a pan, add 1 tbsp oil, garlic and chilli. Saute.
2. Add carrots, baby corn, green beans and cabbage. Saute and add sesame oil. Add the rice.
3. Season with salt and pepper, soy sauce and wine. Cook for a minute.
4. Serve hot garnished with some chopped spring onion greens.

28. Sweet Chicken

Prep Time: 20 Minutes

Cook Time: 1hrs 20 Minutes

Servings: 4

Ingredients

- 1/2 kg boneless chicken (cut as you like it)
- 2 1/2 cups yogurt
- 1 tsp cumin / zeera powder
- 1 tsp garlic paste
- 1/2 tsp red chilli (rang) powder
- A little less than 1/4 tsp turmeric/haldi
- 1/4 tsp garam masala
- Few slit green chillies
- 2 onions, chopped
- 1 tomato, chopped
- Coriander leaves to garnish
- 2 tsp oil
- 1 tsp salt

Instructions

1. Take the yogurt and mix in the cumin powder, garlic paste, garam masala, haldi and red chilli powder. Mix with hands. Put chicken into this and add slit chillies. Keep aside for 30 minutes.
2. Now heat 2 tsp oil in pan and add onions. Cook till translucent and soft.
3. Add the tomatoes. Cook for a minute and add all the chicken and marinade.
4. Keep cooking till gravy reaches the consistency you like. Of you like it more dry, cook a little bit more till yogurt curdles around chicken. Check for salt.
5. Garnish with coriander leaves and enjoy. This can be eaten with rice if the gravy is more and with Indian bread (roti/naan) if you dry it up.

Prep Time: 20 Minutes

Cook Time: 30 Minutes

Servings: 4

Ingredients

- 1/2 Kg Potatoes
- 100 gms Potatoes, mashed
- 100 gms Crumbled paneer
- 1 tsp Red chilli powder and salt
- 1 tsp Garam masala
- 1 1/2 tsp Kasoori methi
- 3 tbsp Ghee
- 1 tbsp Butter
- 1 tbsp Cream

For the onion gravy:

- 200 gms Onions
- 1/2 tsp Garam masala
- to taste Salt
- 1 tsp Ghee

For the tomato gravy:

- 200 gms Fresh tomato puree
- to taste Salt
- 1 tsp Ghee

Instructions

Prepare onion gravy:

1. Heat some ghee in a pan and saute all the ingredients. The onions should be nice and glossy. Keep aside.
2. Prepare tomato gravy:
3. In another pan, heat some ghee and cook all the ingredients for a couple of minutes. Keep aside.

Prepare the potatoes:

1. Cut out the cores of the potatoes and deep fry the potatoes.
2. While the potatoes cool down make the filling. Mix the mashed potatoes and paneer together. This is the filling.
3. Stuff the fried potatoes with the filling and keep aside.

Prepare the final preparation:

1. Cook the onion and tomato gravies in oil until the oil separates.

2. Add all the garama masala, chilli powder and kasoori methi. Mix. Cook for 1 minute.

3. Stir in the butter and the cream. Mix well.4.

4. Finally, add the potatoes and simmer for about 3-5 minutes.

30. Avial with Red Rice

Prep Time: 15 Minutes

Cook Time: 35 Minutes

Servings: 4

Ingredients

For rice:

- 1 cup red rice
- 7 cups water
- For avial:
- 1 potato
- 2 carrots
- 1 raw banana
- 2 drumsticks
- small raw mango (one piece)
- 1 tbsp sour curd
- 5 bean sticks
- 1 large onion
- salt
- 1 tsp turmeric
- 1 cup water

- 1 tbsp coconut oil
- seedless green chillies
- 2 tsp crushed mustard seeds

Instructions

Boil red rice in 7 cups of water for an hour.

Boil potatoes and carrots separately and keep aside.

Take some water in a saucepan. Add chopped raw banana, drumsticks, beans, onion and raw mango.

Then season with salt and turmeric powder. Stir well and let it steam for 2-3 minutes.

Then add green chillies, coconut oil and mustard seeds.

Once the vegetables are steamed, add the boiled potato and carrot along with some curd.

Finally add mustard seeds with coconut oil and mix it well.